27 EASY PANCAKE RECIPES

VALERIE FRETT

AuthorHouse™
1663 Liberty Drive
Bloomington, IN 47403
www.authorhouse.com
Phone: 1 (800) 839-8640

Published by AuthorHouse 06/07/2018

ISBN: 978-1-5462-4264-2 (sc)
ISBN: 978-1-5462-4265-9 (e)

Library of Congress Control Number: 2018906022

Print information available on the last page.

Any people depicted in stock imagery provided by Getty Images are models,
and such images are being used for illustrative purposes only.
Certain stock imagery © Getty Images.

This book is printed on acid-free paper.

Because of the dynamic nature of the Internet, any web addresses or links contained in
this book may have changed since publication and may no longer be valid. The views
expressed in this work are solely those of the author and do not necessarily reflect the views
of the publisher, and the publisher hereby disclaims any responsibility for them.

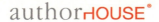

Contents

Acknowledgement

I received great help from some very kind people and I would like to thank them; Mae Genson, my publishing consultant, for her continuous support and guidance; Shawn and Sheldon Frett and Shawnea Frett Ajao for assistance in organizing my work.

Introduction

When it comes to sugar and sweetness, persons have individual tastes and preferences. Some people like more or less sweetness than others. For that matter, persons using these recipes can slightly alter the amount of sugar they use. Persons can also substitute other types of sweeteners for sugar. For example, if one prefers, one may use honey or agave, or any of the other sweeteners in place of sugar. For persons with diabetes or with a glucose level that tends to be elevated, they can substitute sugar with stevia, which is a sweetner from plant that has a minimal amount of calories.

Each packet of Stevia in the Raw has the sweetness of 2 teaspoons of sugar and is 1 gram in volume. Therefore, 1 gram of Stevia in the Raw equals 2 teaspoons of sugar.

Similarly, persons can substitute their favorite oil. There are so many different ones.

Persons who are sensitive to gluten can substitute their preferred flour, for example Buckwheat or any gluten free flour. A little tapioca flour or arrowroot can help to bind any flour that doesn't hold together well.

Make your own pancake mix and avoid all the preservatives and additives of on-the-shelf pancake mixes. Individuals can use their preferred ingredients for custom-made pancakes. Those covered in this book are not an exhaustive list of pancakes. Rather, they can stimulate ideas and combinations of your own.

How to Cook a Pancake

Heat a non-stick griddle over medium heat.
Pour pancake mixture in a circle about 5 inches in diameter.
Cook pancake until little bubbles appear, about 5 minutes.
Turn pancake with a spatula onto its other side.
Cook until the inside is done, about 4 minutes.
Remove pancake from griddle.

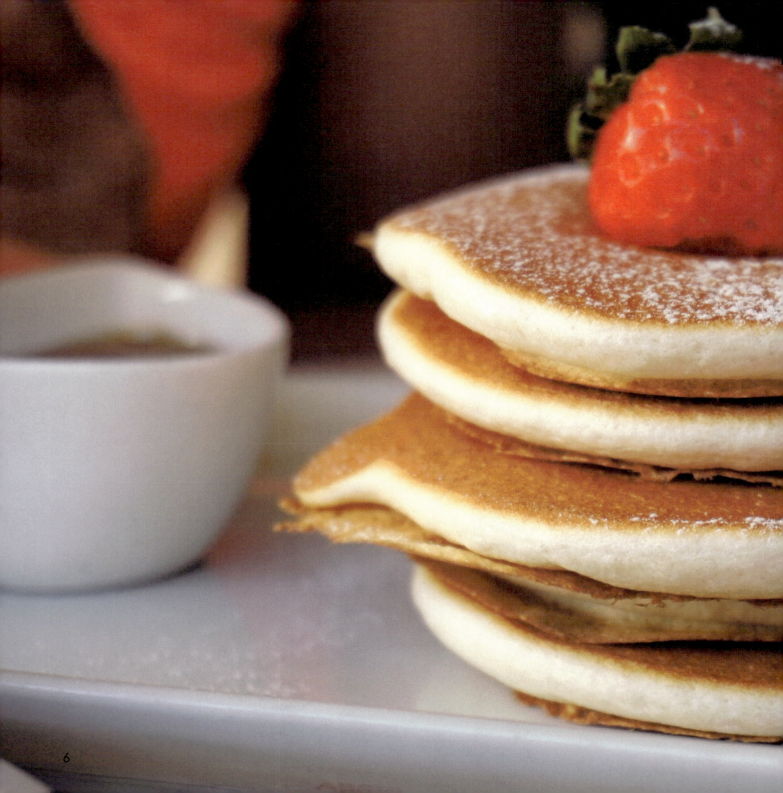

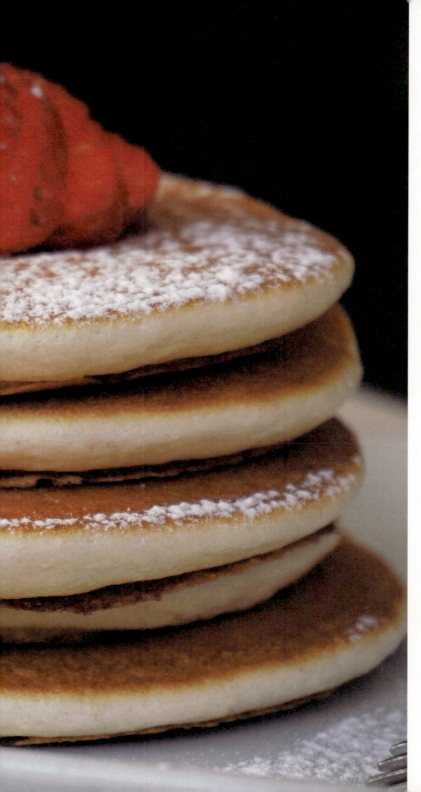

Plain Pancake

Ingredients

2 large eggs
A pinch of salt
½ teaspoon baking powder
½ teaspoon grated nutmeg
1 teaspoon ground cinnamon
1 teaspoon vanilla
1 tablespoon sugar
¼ cup olive oil
¼ cup milk (optional)
1/3 or ½ cup all-purpose flour

Method

Beat eggs well.
Add salt, sugar and spices. Beat.
Add olive oil. Beat.
(Add milk. Beat.)
Fold in 1/3 cup flour and baking
powder without milk.
Or fold in ½ cup flour and
baking powder with milk.
Cook pancakes in the usual way.

Makes 3 to 4 medium size pancakes.

Flavored Pancake

Ingredients

2 large eggs
A pinch of salt
½ teaspoon baking powder
½ teaspoon grated nutmeg
1 teaspoon ground cinnamon
1 teaspoon vanilla
1 tablespoon sugar
¼ cup olive oil
¼ cup any fruit or vegetable juice
½ cup all-purpose flour

Method

Beat eggs well.
Add salt, sugar and spices. Beat.
Add olive oil. Beat.
Add juice. Beat.
Fold in flour and baking powder.
Cook pancakes in the usual way.

Makes 4 medium size pancakes.

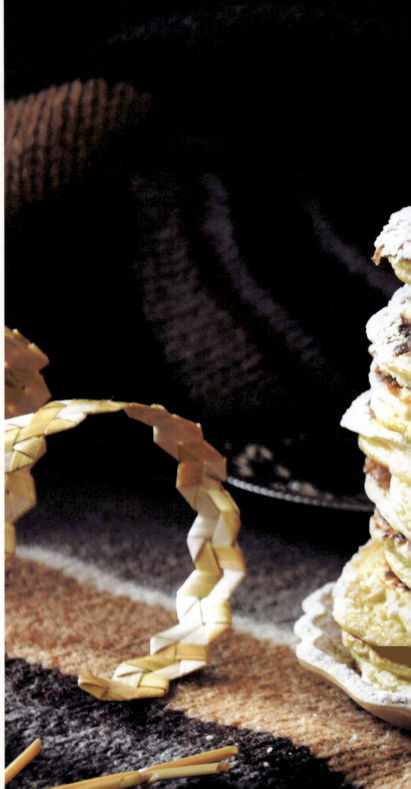

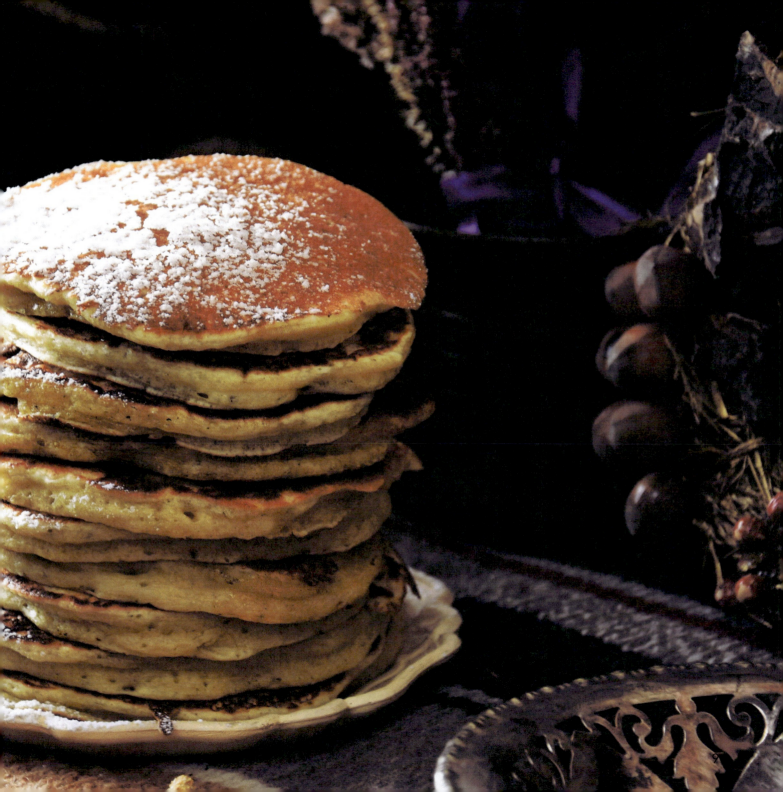

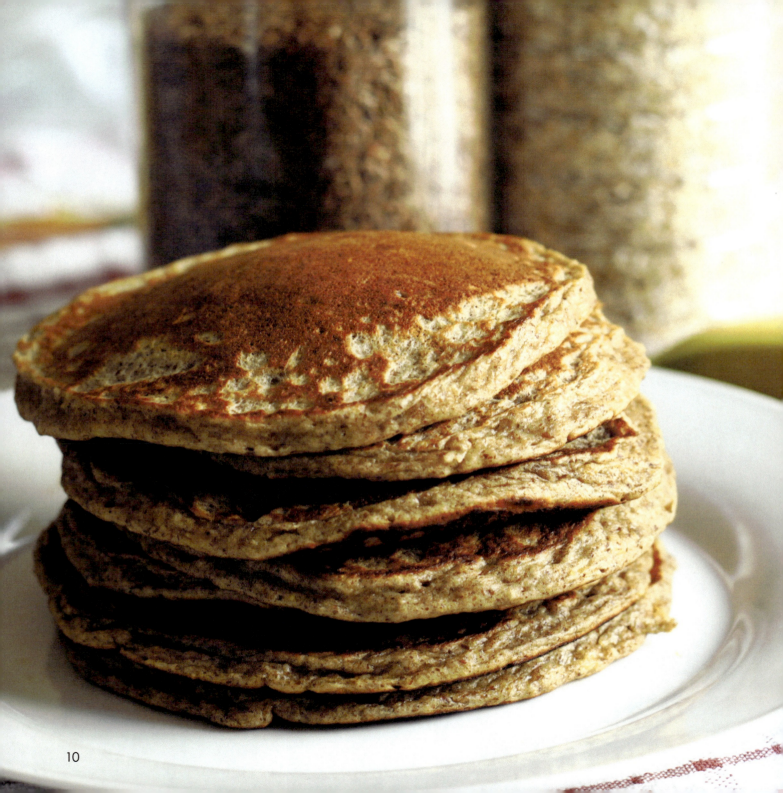

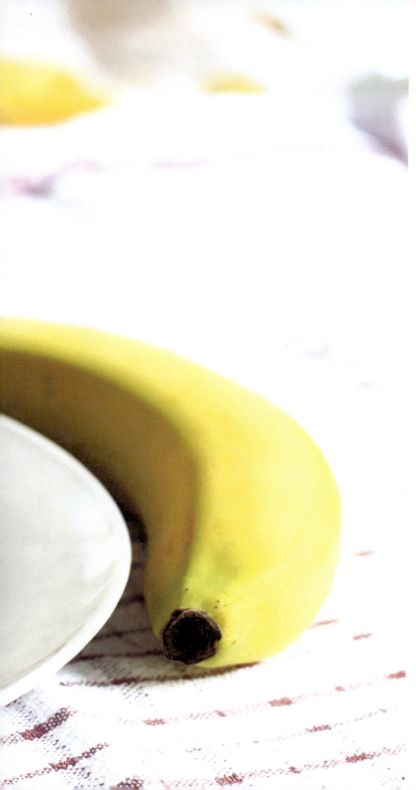

Banana Pancake

Ingredients

2 large eggs
2 medium size very ripe bananas
A pinch of salt
½ teaspoon baking powder (optional)
½ teaspoon grated nutmeg
1 teaspoon ground cinnamon
1 teaspoon vanilla
1 tablespoon sugar
3 tablespoon olive oil
½ cup all-purpose flour

Method

Mash bananas to a paste.
Beat eggs well.
Add beaten eggs to bananas. Beat.
Add salt, sugar and spices. Beat.
Add olive oil. Beat.
Fold in flour (and baking powder).
Cook pancakes in the usual way.

Makes 4 medium size pancakes.

Oatmeal Pancake

Ingredients

2 large eggs
A pinch of salt
½ teaspoon baking powder
½ teaspoon grated nutmeg
1 teaspoon ground cinnamon
1 teaspoon vanilla
1 tablespoon sugar
¼ cup olive oil
¼ cup all-purpose flour
1/3 cup quick 1-minute oatmeal

Method

Beat eggs well.
Add salt, sugar and spices. Beat.
Add olive oil. Beat.
Fold in oatmeal.
Fold in flour and baking powder.
Cook pancakes in the usual way.

Makes 3 medium size pancakes.

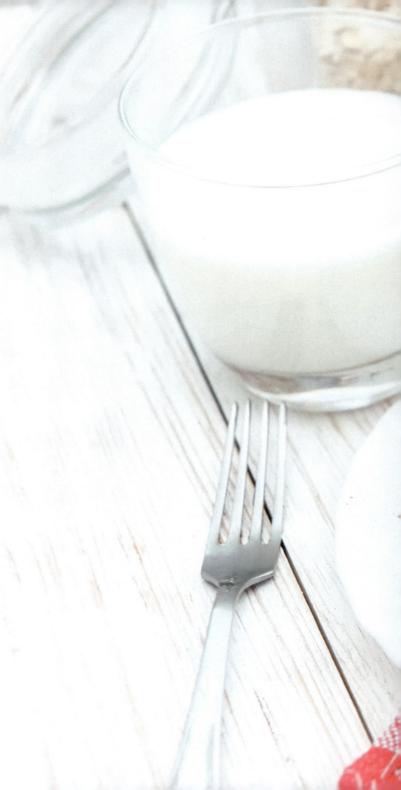

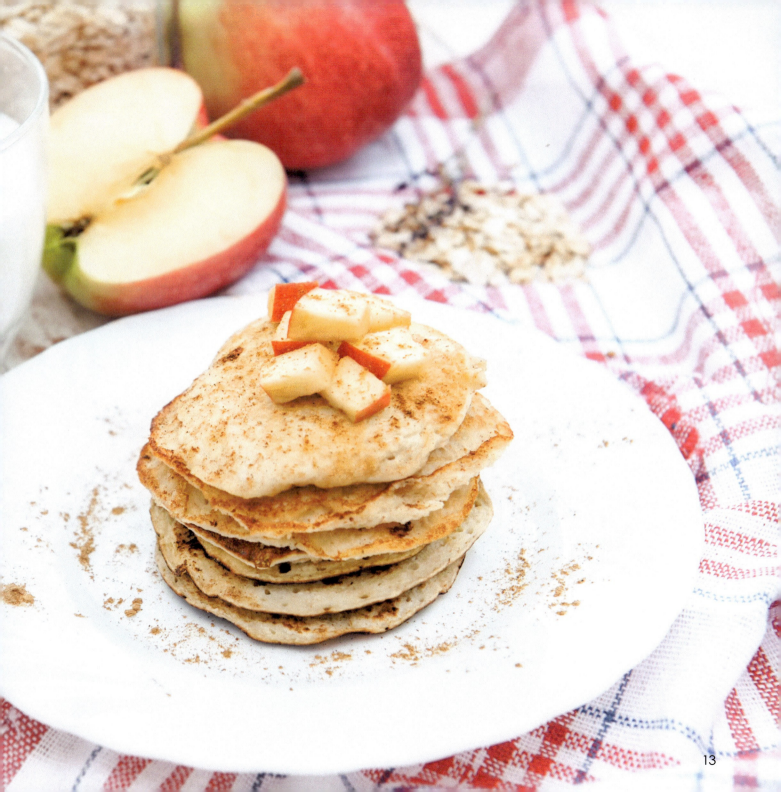

Blueberry Pancake

Ingredients

2 large eggs
A pinch of salt
½ teaspoon baking powder
½ teaspoon grated nutmeg
1 teaspoon cinnamon
1 teaspoon vanilla
1 tablespoon sugar
¼ cup olive oil
1/3 cup all-purpose flour
½ cup small, fresh blueberries

Method

Rinse and pat dry blueberries on paper towel.
Beat eggs well.
Add salt, sugar and spices. Beat.
Add olive oil. Beat.
Mix in blueberries.
Fold in flour and baking powder.
Cook pancakes in the usual way.

Makes 3 medium size pancakes.

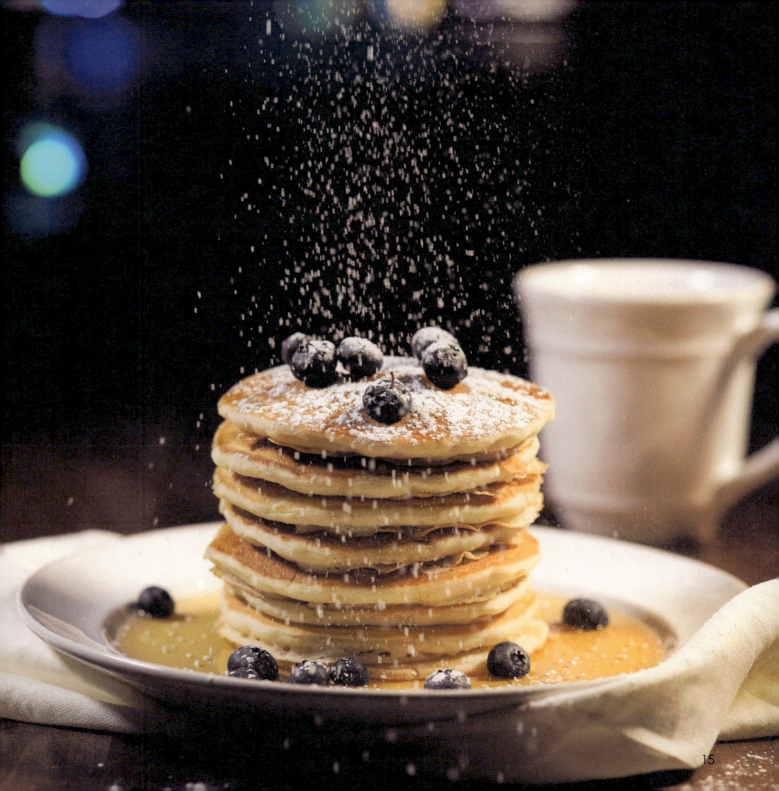

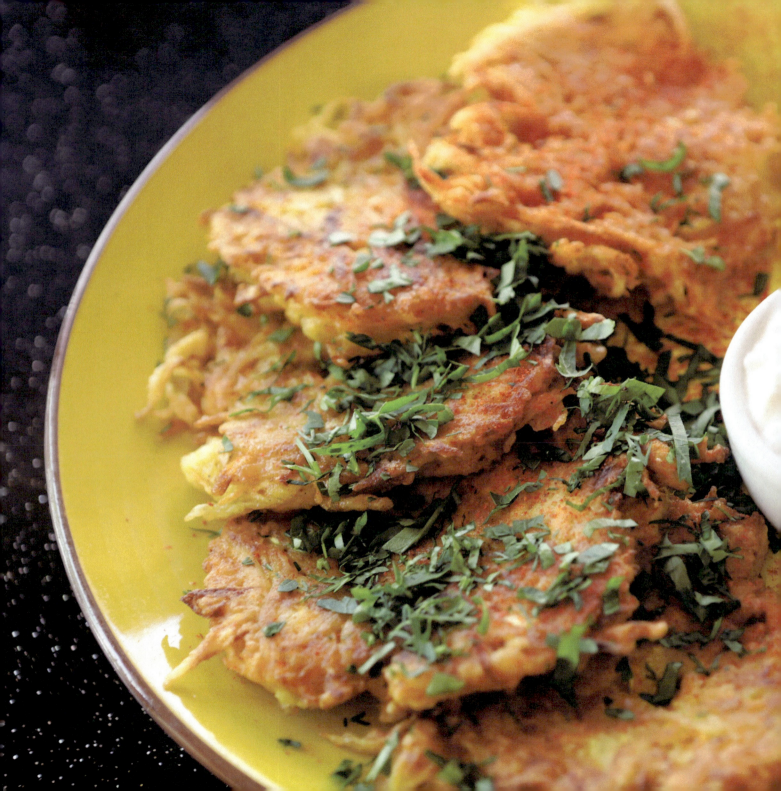

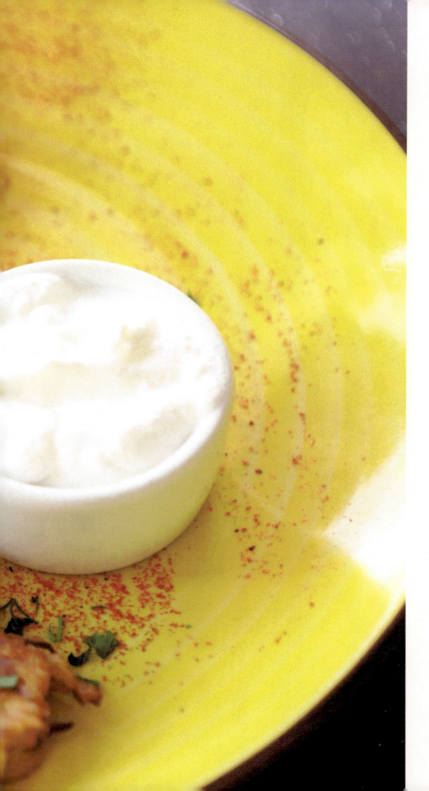

Carrot Pancake

Ingredients

2 large eggs
A pinch of salt
½ teaspoon baking powder
½ teaspoon grated nutmeg
1 teaspoon ground cinnamon
1 teaspoon vanilla
1 tablespoon sugar
¼ cup olive oil
1/3 cup all-purpose flour
¾ cup grated carrot or
cooked, mashed carrot

Method

Beat eggs well.
Add salt, sugar and spices. Beat.
Add olive oil. Beat.
Mix in carrot.
Fold in flour and baking powder.
Cook pancakes in the usual way.

Makes 3 medium size pancakes.

Sweet Potato Pancake

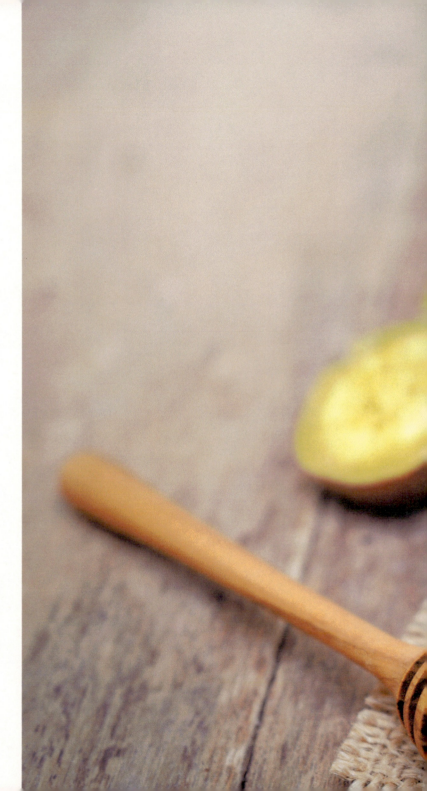

Ingredients

2 large eggs
A pinch of salt
½ teaspoon baking powder
½ teaspoon grated nutmeg
1 teaspoon ground cinnamon
1 teaspoon vanilla
1 tablespoon sugar
¼ cup olive oil
¼ cup all-purpose flour
¾ cup grated sweet potato

Method

Beat eggs well.
Add salt, sugar and spices. Beat.
Add olive oil. Beat.
Mix in sweet potato.
Fold in flour and baking powder.
Cook pancakes in the usual way.

Makes 3 medium size pancakes.

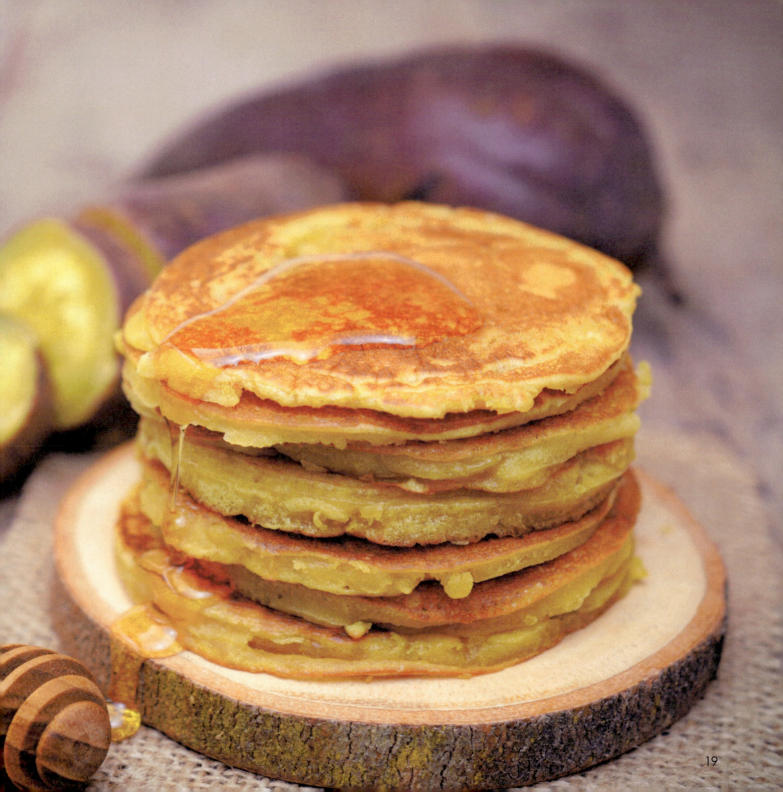

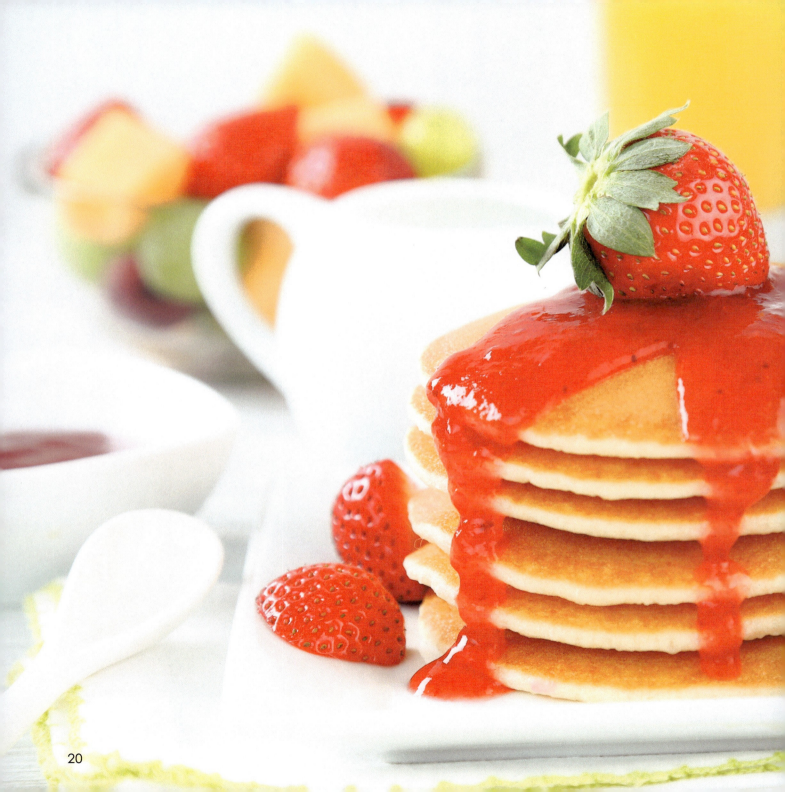

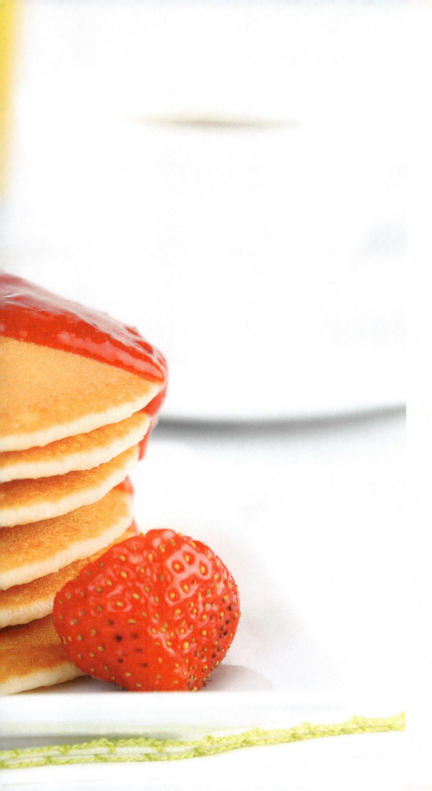

Strawberry Pancake

Ingredients

2 large eggs
A pinch of salt
½ teaspoon baking powder
½ teaspoon grated nutmeg
1 teaspoon ground cinnamon
1 teaspoon vanilla
1 tablespoon sugar
¼ cup olive oil
1/3 cup all-purpose flour
½ cup fresh strawberries cut up
into small cubes or thinly sliced

Method

Beat eggs well.
Add salt, sugar and spices. Beat.
Add olive oil. Beat.
Mix in strawberries.
Fold in flour and baking powder.
Cook pancakes in the usual way.

Makes 2 medium size pancakes.

Zucchini Pancake

Ingredients

2 large eggs
A pinch of salt
½ teaspoon baking powder
½ teaspoon grated nutmeg
1 teaspoon ground cinnamon
1 teaspoon vanilla
2 tablespoon sugar
¼ cup olive oil
1/3 cup all-purpose flour
1 small zucchini grated

Method

Beat eggs well.
Add salt, sugar and spices. Beat.
Add olive oil. Beat.
Add zucchini. Beat.
Fold in flour and baking powder.
Cook pancakes in the usual way.

Makes 3 to 4 medium size pancakes.

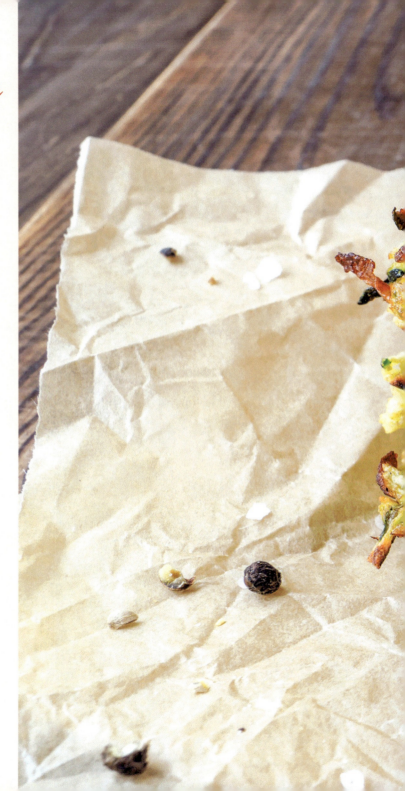

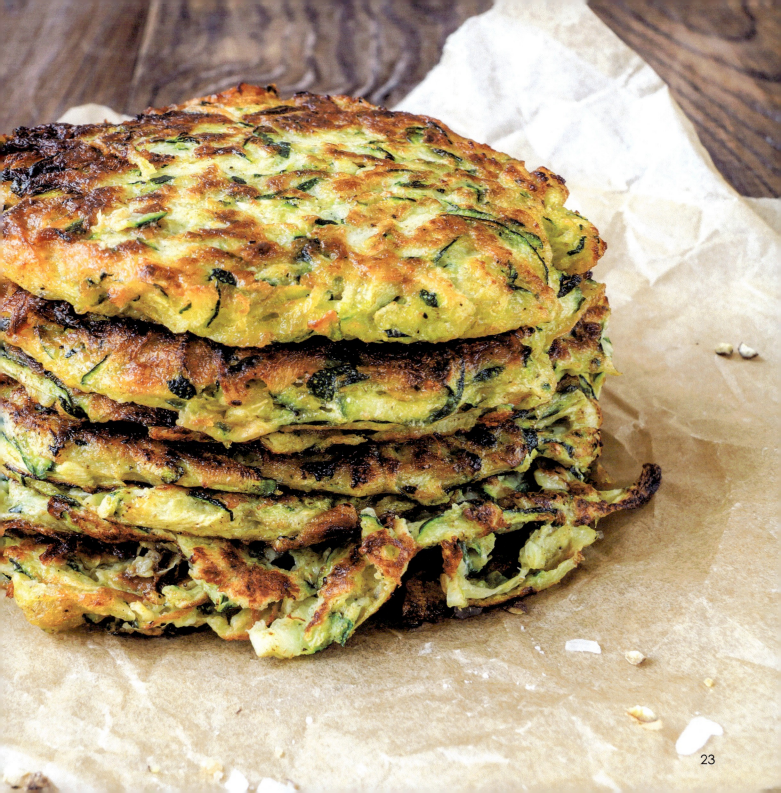

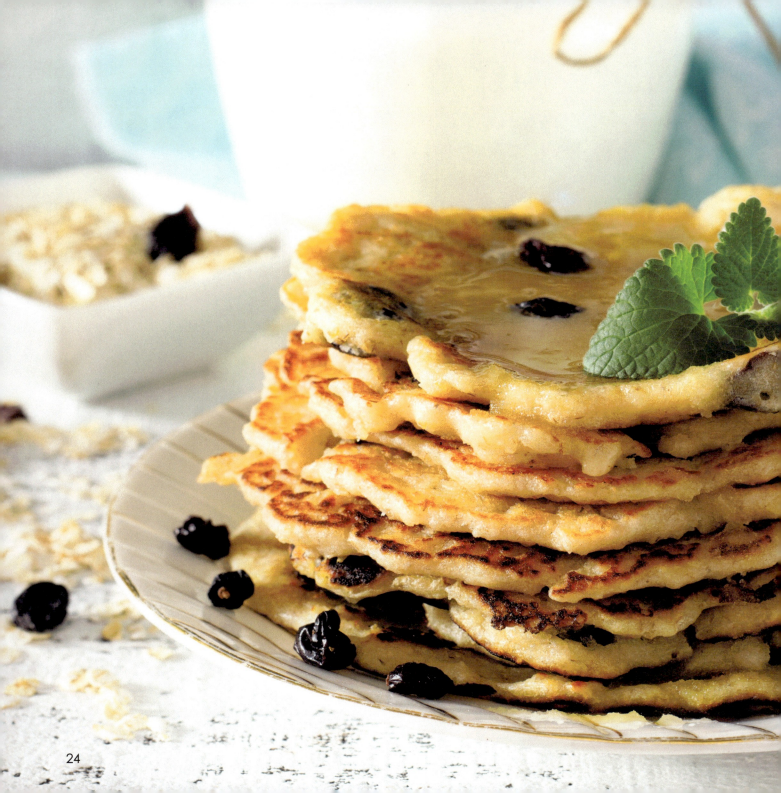

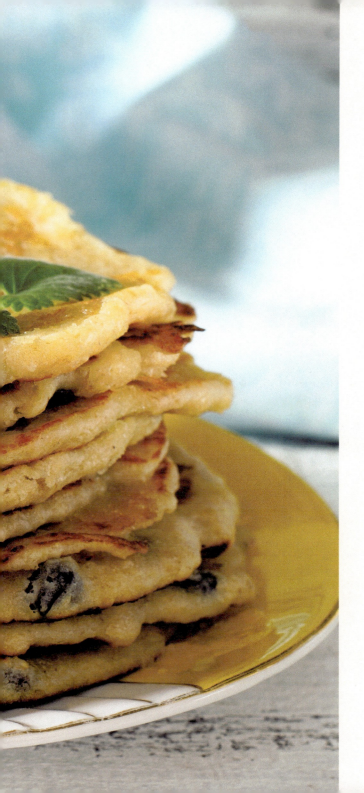

Oatmeal Raisin Pancake

Ingredients

2 large eggs
A pinch of salt
½ teaspoon baking powder
½ teaspoon grated nutmeg
1 teaspoon ground cinnamon
1 teaspoon vanilla
1 tablespoon sugar
¼ cup olive oil
¼ cup raisins
¼ cup all-purpose flour
1/3 cup quick 1-minute oatmeal

Method

Beat eggs well.
Add salt, sugar and spices. Beat.
Add olive oil. Beat.
Fold in oatmeal and raisins.
Fold in flour and baking powder.
Cook pancakes in the usual way.

Makes 3 medium size pancakes.

Cinnamon Raisin Pancake

Ingredients

2 large eggs
A pinch of salt
½ teaspoon baking powder
½ teaspoon grated nutmeg
1 teaspoon vanilla
2 teaspoon ground cinnamon
1 tablespoon sugar
¼ cup olive oil
¼ cup raisins
1/3 cup all-purpose flour

Method

Beat eggs well.
Add salt, sugar and spices. Beat.
Add olive oil. Beat.
Mix in raisins.
Fold in flour and baking powder.
Cook pancakes in the usual way.

Makes 2 medium size pancakes.

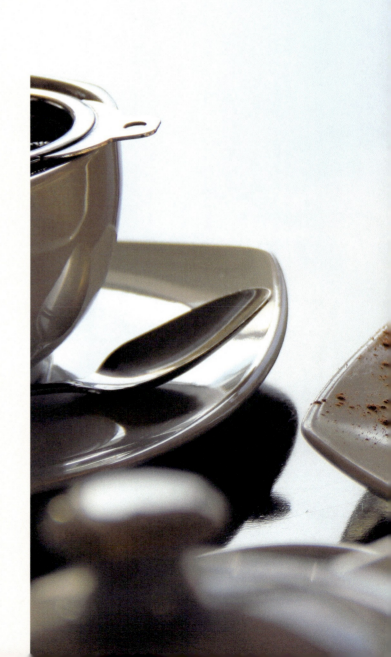

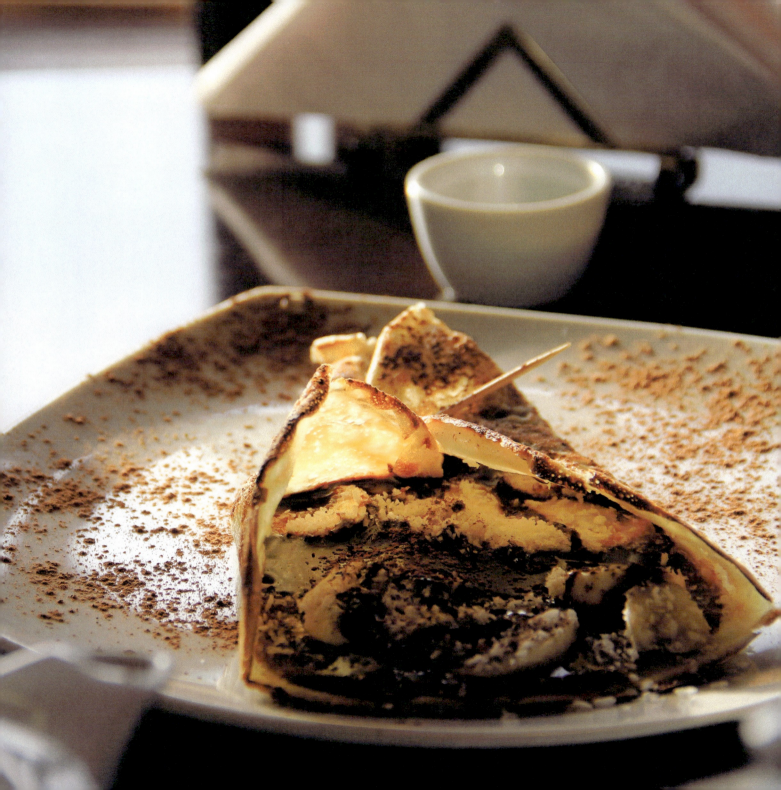

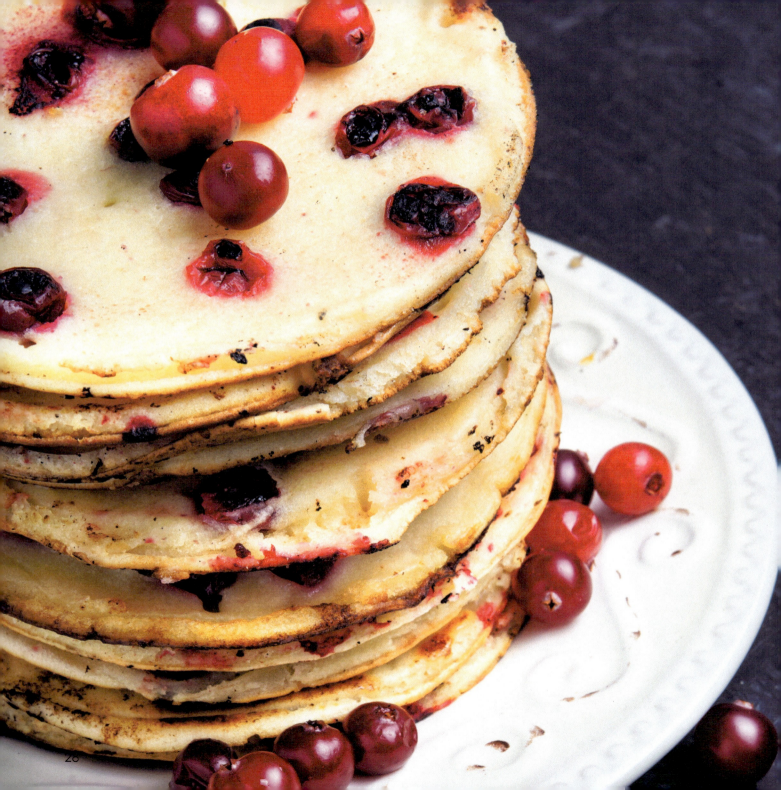

Cranberry Pancake

Ingredients

2 large eggs
A pinch of salt
½ teaspoon baking powder
½ teaspoon grated nutmeg
1 teaspoon ground cinnamon
1 teaspoon vanilla
1 tablespoon sugar
¼ cup olive oil
1/3 cup dried cranberries
1/3 cup all-purpose flour

Method

Beat eggs well.
Add salt, sugar and spices. Beat.
Add olive oil. Beat.
Mix in cranberries.
Fold in flour and baking powder.
Cook pancakes in the usual way.

Makes 2 medium size pancakes.

Cornmeal Pancake

Ingredients

2 large eggs
A pinch of salt
½ teaspoon baking powder
½ teaspoon grated nutmeg
1 teaspoon ground cinnamon
1 teaspoon vanilla
1 tablespoon sugar
¼ cup olive oil
¼ cup medium ground cornmeal
¼ cup all-purpose flour

Method

Cook cornmeal and salt in ¾ cup
water for 10 minutes on low fire,
stirring frequently. Let cool.
Beat eggs well.
Add sugar and spices. Beat.
Add olive oil. Beat.
Add cooked cornmeal. Beat.
Fold in flour and baking powder.
Cook pancakes in the usual way.

Makes 3 medium size pancakes.

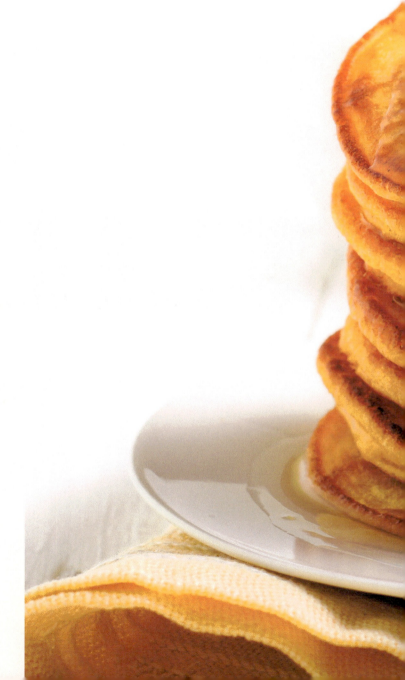

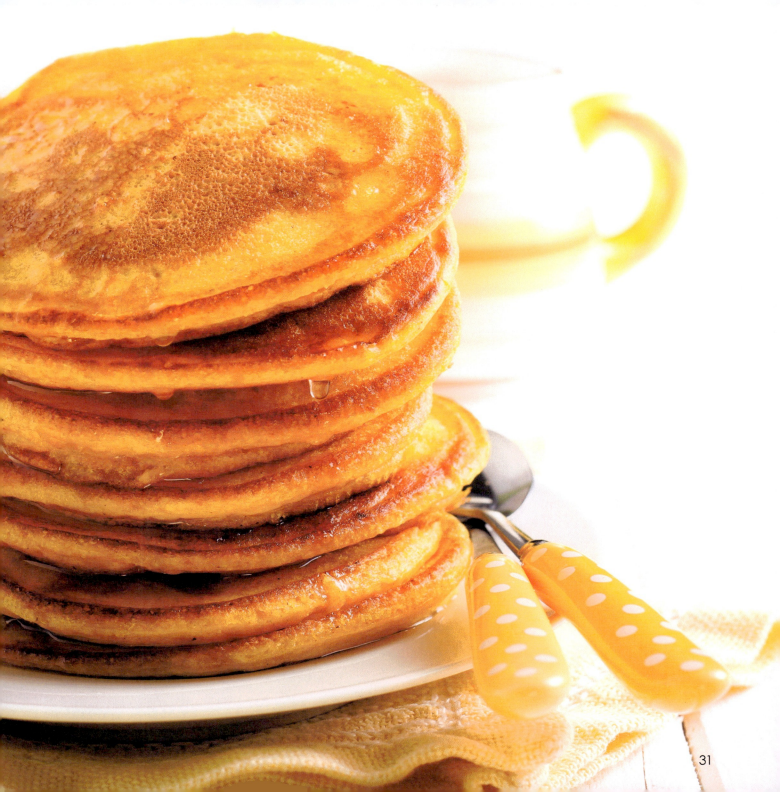

Whole Wheat Pancake

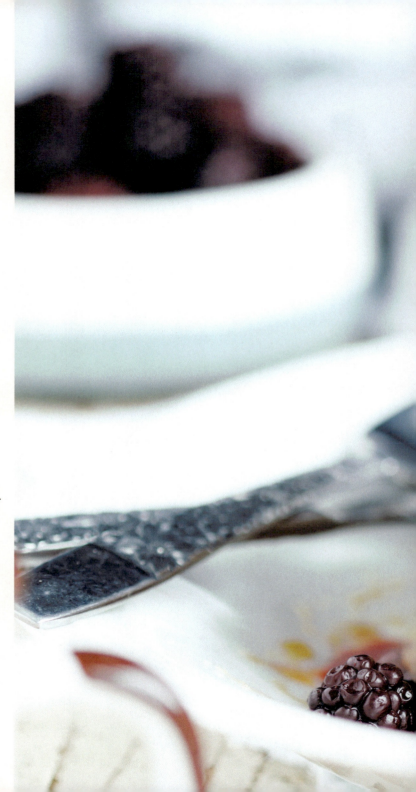

Ingredients

2 large eggs
A pinch of salt
½ teaspoon baking powder
½ teaspoon grated nutmeg
1 teaspoon ground cinnamon
1 teaspoon vanilla
1 tablespoon sugar
¼ cup olive oil
¼ cup whole grain cracked wheat
¼ cup all-purpose flour

Method

Cook cracked wheat in ½ cup water
for 10 minutes on low fire. Let cool.
Beat eggs well.
Add salt, sugar and spices. Beat.
Add olive oil. Beat.
Add cooked wheat. Beat.
Fold in flour and baking powder.
Cook pancakes in the usual way.

Makes 3 medium size pancakes.

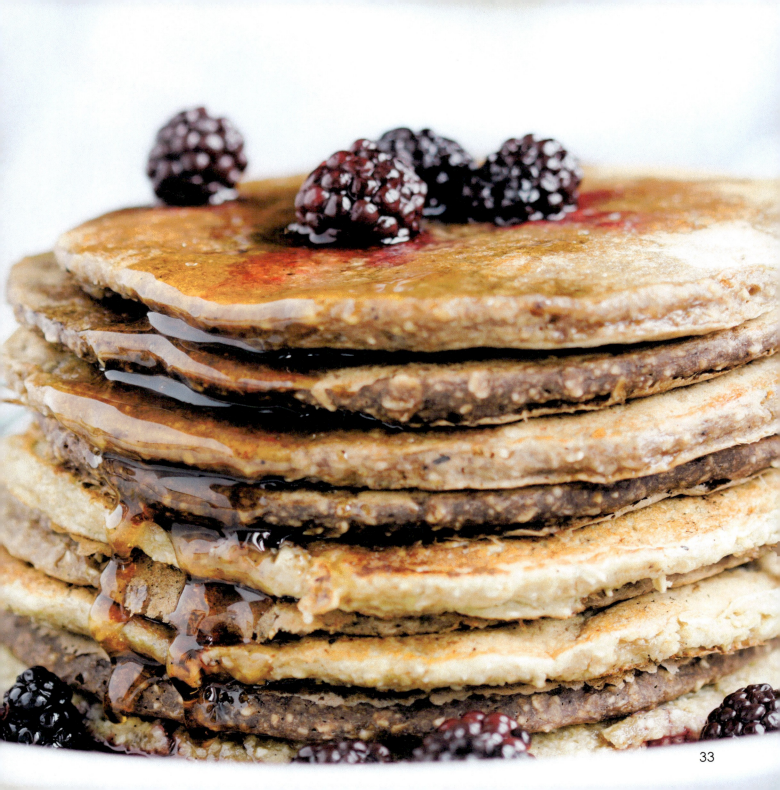

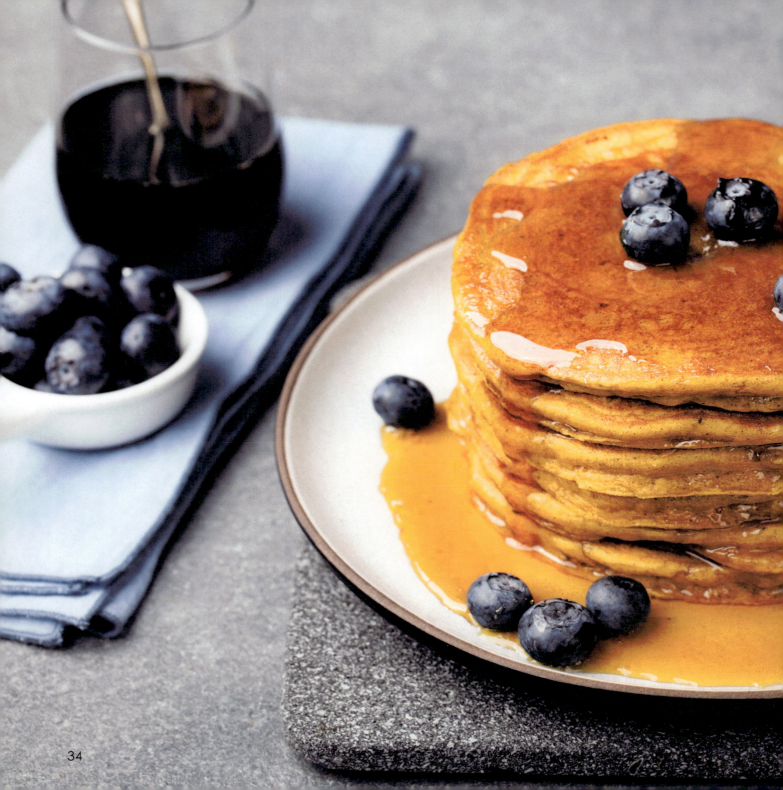

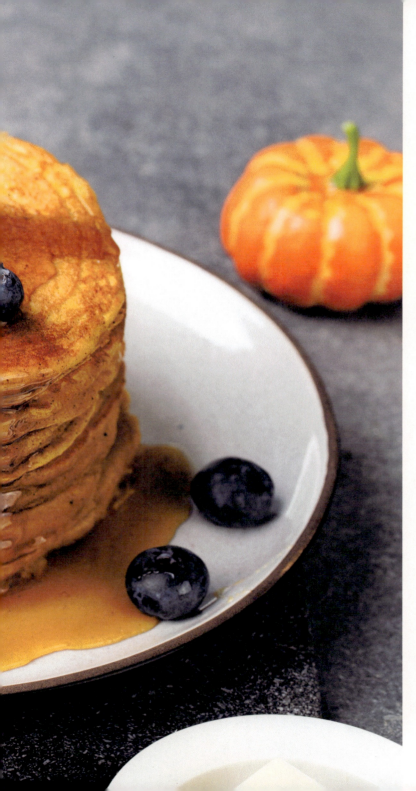

Pumpkin Pancake

Ingredients

2 large eggs
A pinch of salt
½ teaspoon baking powder
½ teaspoon grated nutmeg
1 teaspoon ground cinnamon
1 teaspoon vanilla
1 tablespoon sugar
¼ cup olive oil
1/3 cup all-purpose flour
¾ cup grated or ½ cup cooked
and mashed pumpkin

Method

Beat eggs well.
Add salt, sugar and spices. Beat.
Add olive oil. Beat.
Add ½ cup cooked and
mashed pumpkin. Beat.
Or
Mix in ¾ cup grated pumpkin.
Fold in flour and baking powder.
Cook pancakes in the usual way.

Makes 3 to 4 medium size pancakes.

Pineapple Pancake

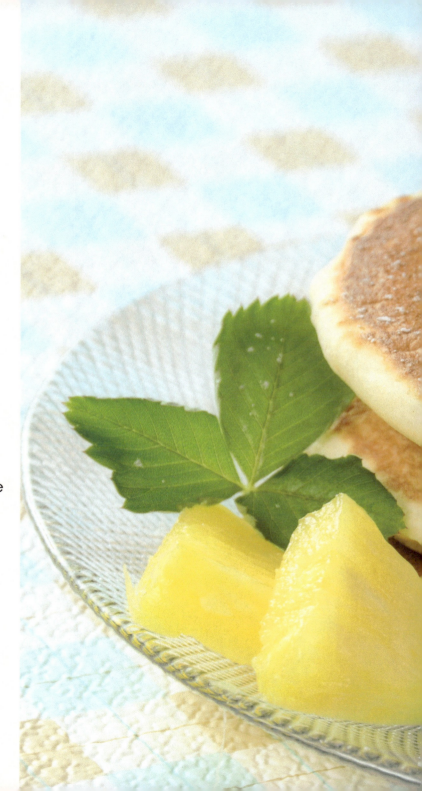

Ingredients

2 large eggs
A pinch of salt
½ teaspoon baking powder
½ teaspoon grated nutmeg
1 teaspoon ground cinnamon
1 teaspoon vanilla
1 tablespoon sugar
¼ cup olive oil
1/3 cup all-purpose flour
½ cup crushed, canned
pineapple drained
or
¾ cup cubed small, fresh pineapple

Method

Beat eggs well.
Add salt, sugar and spices. Beat.
Add olive oil. Beat.
Mix in pineapple.
Fold in flour and baking powder.
Cook pancakes in the usual way.

Makes 3 medium size pancakes.

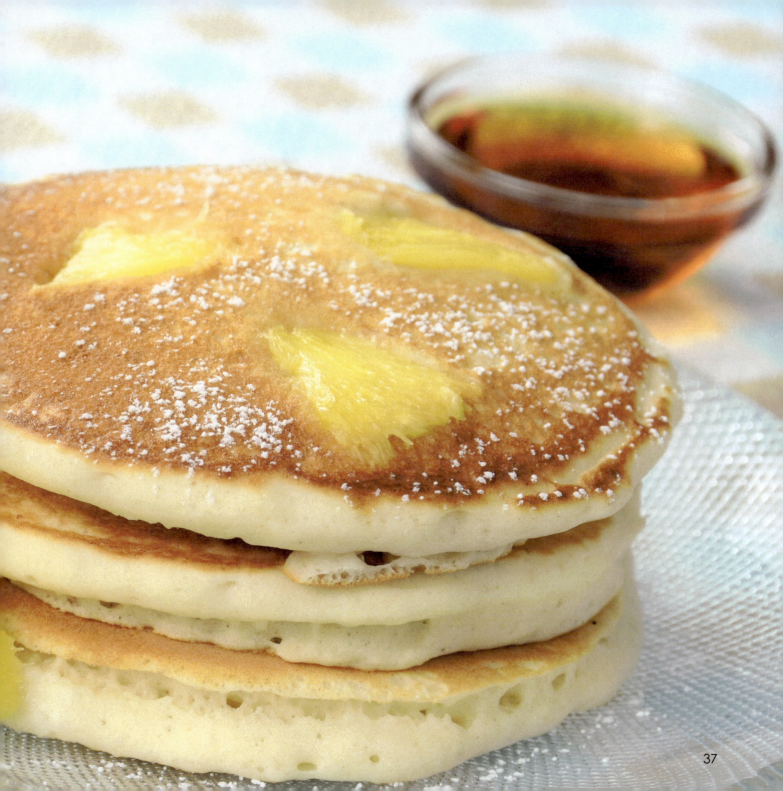

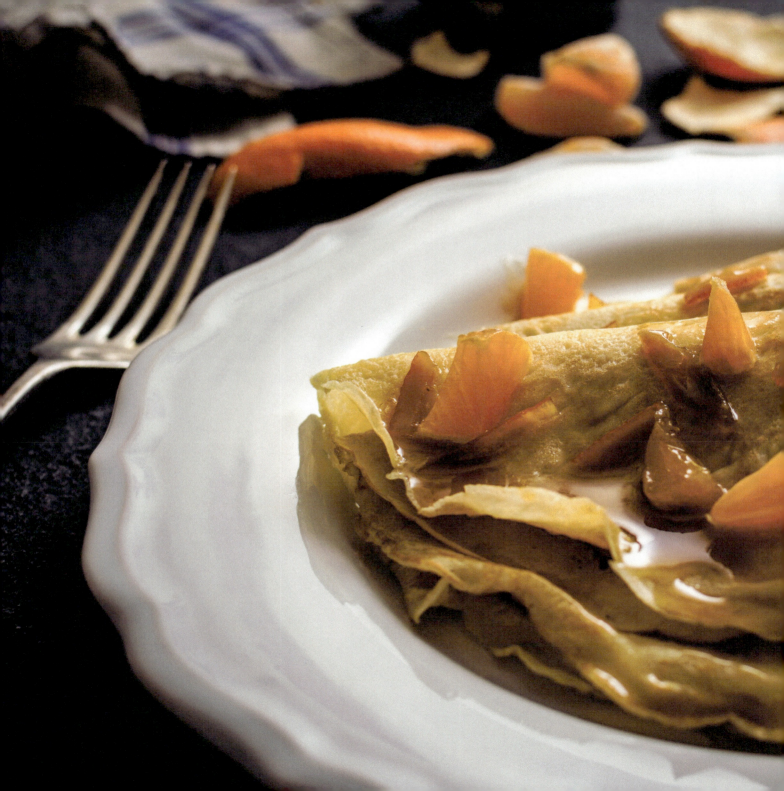

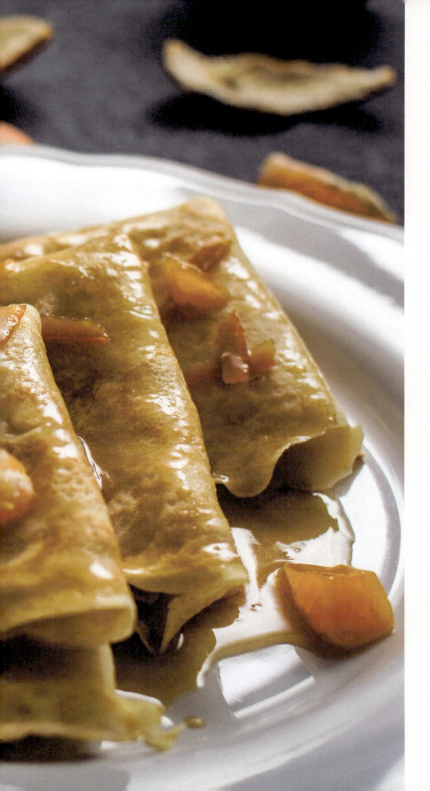

Mandarin Pancake

Ingredients

2 large eggs
A pinch of salt
½ teaspoon baking powder
½ teaspoon grated nutmeg
1 teaspoon ground cinnamon
1 teaspoon vanilla
1 tablespoon sugar
¼ cup olive oil
½ cup all-purpose flour
½ cup drained mandarin
orange pulps from can

Method

Beat eggs well.
Add salt, sugar and spices. Beat.
Add olive oil. Beat.
Mix in mandarin orange pulps.
Fold in flour and baking powder.
Cook pancakes in the usual way.

Makes 3 medium size pancakes.

Fresh Orange Pancake

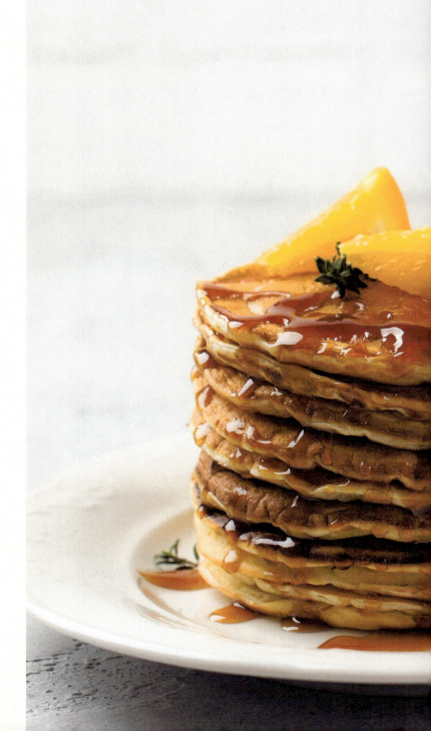

Ingredients

2 large eggs
A pinch of salt
½ teaspoon baking powder
½ teaspoon grated nutmeg
1 teaspoon ground cinnamon
1 teaspoon vanilla
1 tablespoon sugar
¼ cup olive oil
½ cup fresh orange pulps
1/3 cup all-purpose flour

Method

Beat eggs well.
Add salt, sugar and spices. Beat.
Add olive oil. Beat.
Mix in orange pulps.
Fold in flour and baking powder.
Cook pancakes in the usual way.

Makes 3 medium size pancakes.

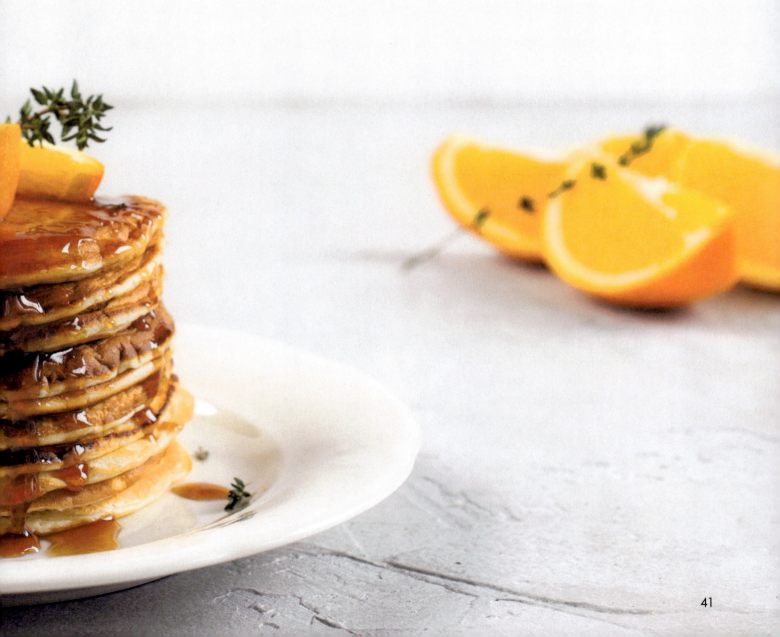

Spinach Pancake

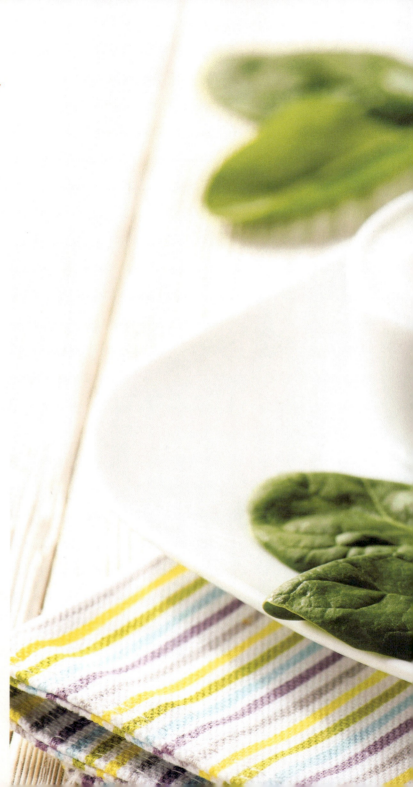

Ingredients

2 large eggs
A pinch of salt
½ teaspoon baking powder
½ teaspoon grated nutmeg
1 teaspoon ground cinnamon
1 teaspoon vanilla
2 tablespoon sugar
¼ cup olive oil
1/3 cup all-purpose flour
¾ cup chopped, fresh spinach
Or ½ cup frozen chopped
spinach thawed and drained

Method

Beat eggs well.
Add salt, sugar and spices. Beat.
Add olive oil. Beat.
Mix in spinach.
Fold in flour and baking powder.
An extra tablespoon of flour may be
needed for thawed, frozen spinach.
Cook pancakes in the usual way.

Makes 2 to 3 medium size pancakes.

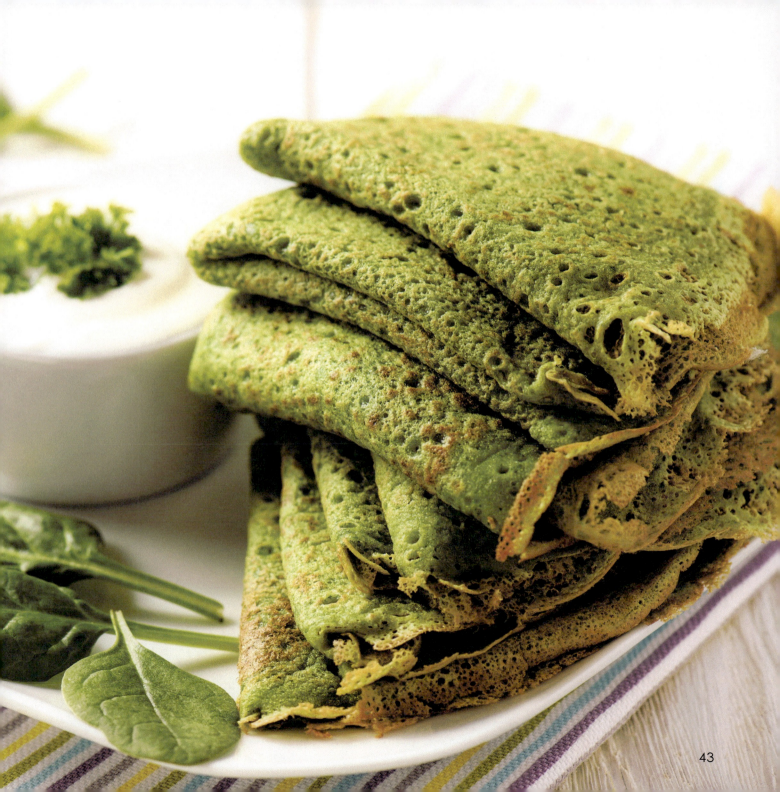

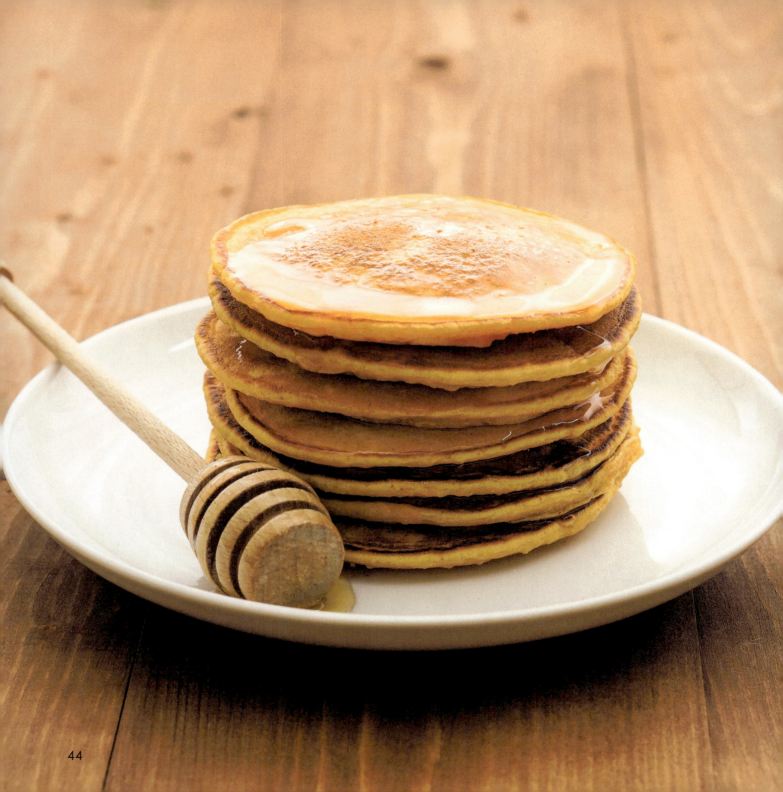

Butternut Pancake

Ingredients

2 large eggs
A pinch of salt
½ teaspoon baking powder
½ teaspoon grated nutmeg
1 teaspoon ground cinnamon
1 teaspoon vanilla
1 tablespoon sugar
¼ cup olive oil
1/3 cup all-purpose flour
½ cup cooked and mashed or ¾ cup grated butternut squash

Method

Beat eggs well.
Add salt, sugar and spices. Beat.
Add olive oil. Beat.
Add cooked and mashed butternut squash. Beat.
Or mix in grated butternut squash.
Fold in flour and baking powder.
Cook pancakes in the usual way.

Makes 3 to 4 medium size pancakes.

Granola Pancake

Ingredients

2 large eggs
A pinch of salt
½ teaspoon baking powder
½ teaspoon grated nutmeg
1 teaspoon ground cinnamon
1 teaspoon vanilla
1 tablespoon sugar
¼ cup olive oil
1/3 cup all-purpose flour
½ cup granola

Method

Beat eggs well.
Add salt, sugar and spices. Beat.
Add olive oil. Beat.
Mix in granola.
Fold in flour and baking powder.
Cook pancakes in the usual way.

Makes 3 medium size pancakes.

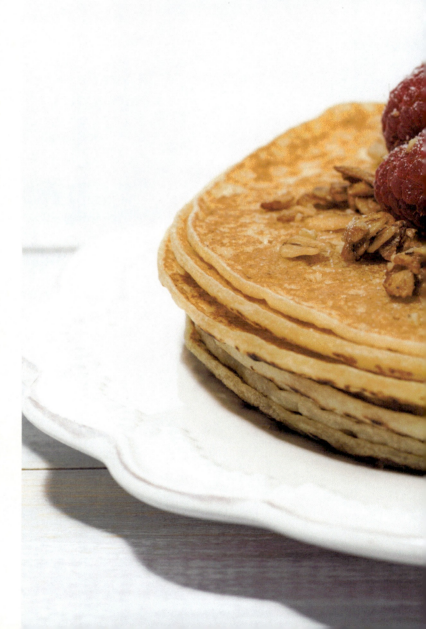

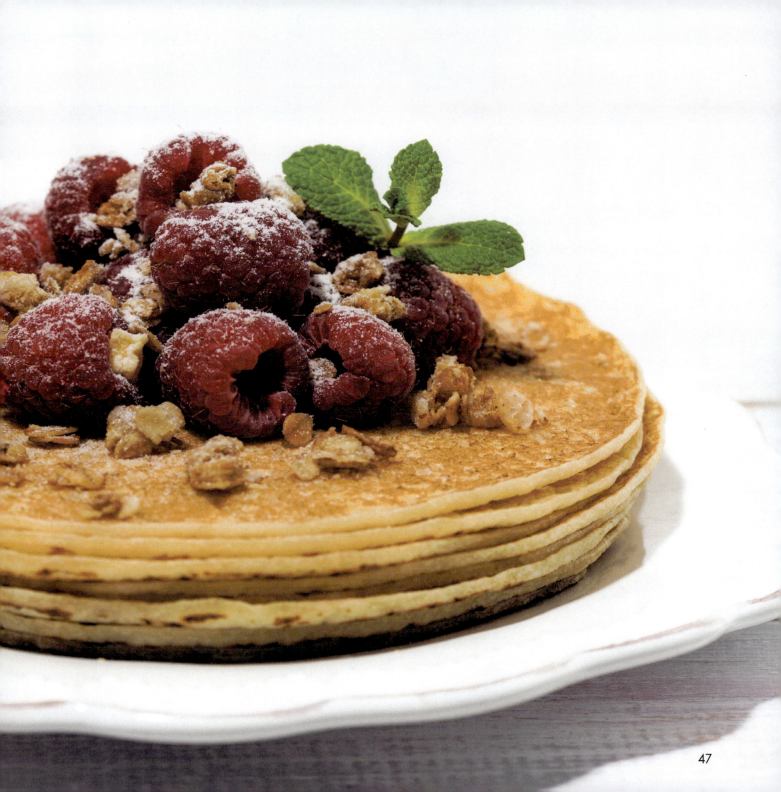

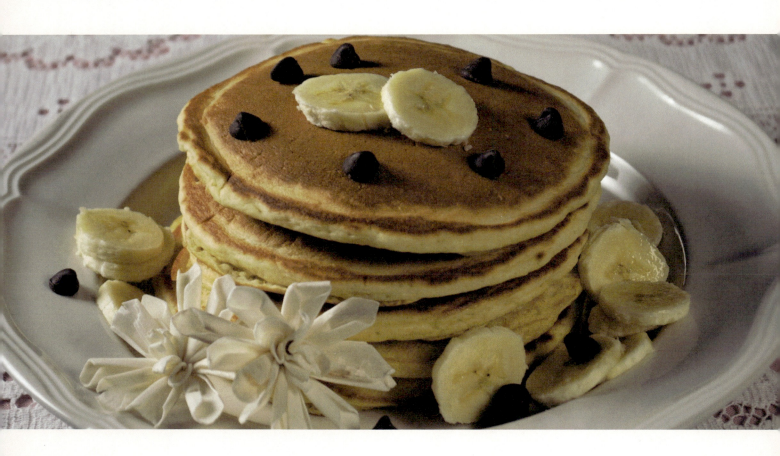

Chocolate Chip Pancake

Ingredients

2 large eggs
A pinch of salt
½ teaspoon baking powder
½ teaspoon grated nutmeg
1 teaspoon ground cinnamon
1 teaspoon vanilla
1 tablespoon sugar
¼ cup olive oil
¼ to ½ cup chocolate chips according to preference
1/3 cup all-purpose flour

Method

Beat eggs well.
Add salt, sugar and spices. Beat.
Add olive oil. Beat.
Mix in chocolate chips.
Fold in flour and baking powder.
Cook pancakes in the usual way.

Makes 3 medium size pancakes.

Raisin Bran Pancake

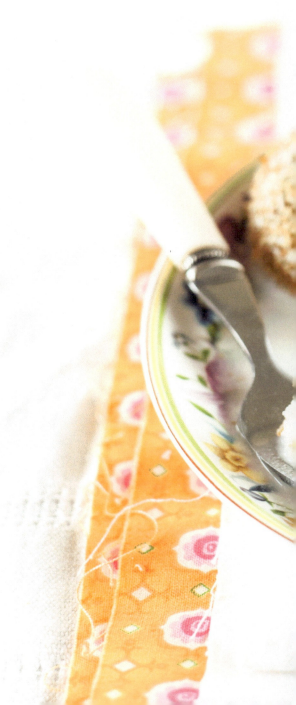

Ingredients

2 large eggs
A pinch of salt
½ teaspoon baking powder
½ teaspoon grated nutmeg
1 teaspoon ground cinnamon
1 teaspoon vanilla
1 tablespoon sugar
¼ cup olive oil
1/3 cup all-purpose flour
1 cup raisin bran

Method

Beat eggs well.
Add salt, sugar and spices. Beat.
Add olive oil. Beat.
Mix in raisin bran.
Fold in flour and baking powder.
Cook pancakes in the usual way.

Makes 3 medium size pancakes.

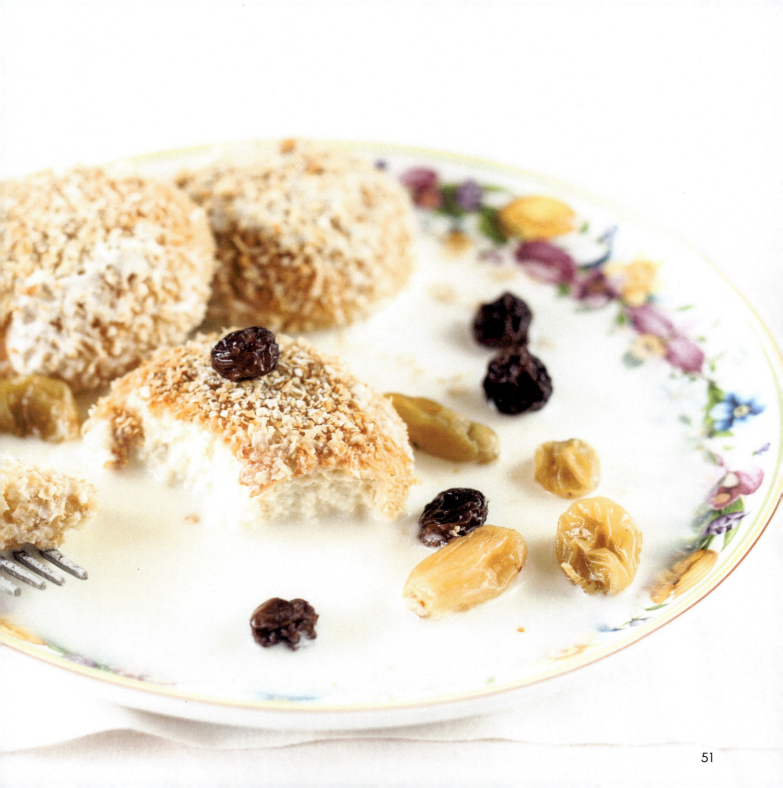

Savory Pancakes

If you are an avid pancake lover, you will also love savory pancakes. Any one of the vegetable pancakes can be made savory by eliminating the sugar and adding your favorite seasonings with enough salt for flavor.

After you have tried the savory pancakes in this book, you will be inspired to create a variety of more savory pancakes of your own liking.

Have a happy experience of pancake creations.

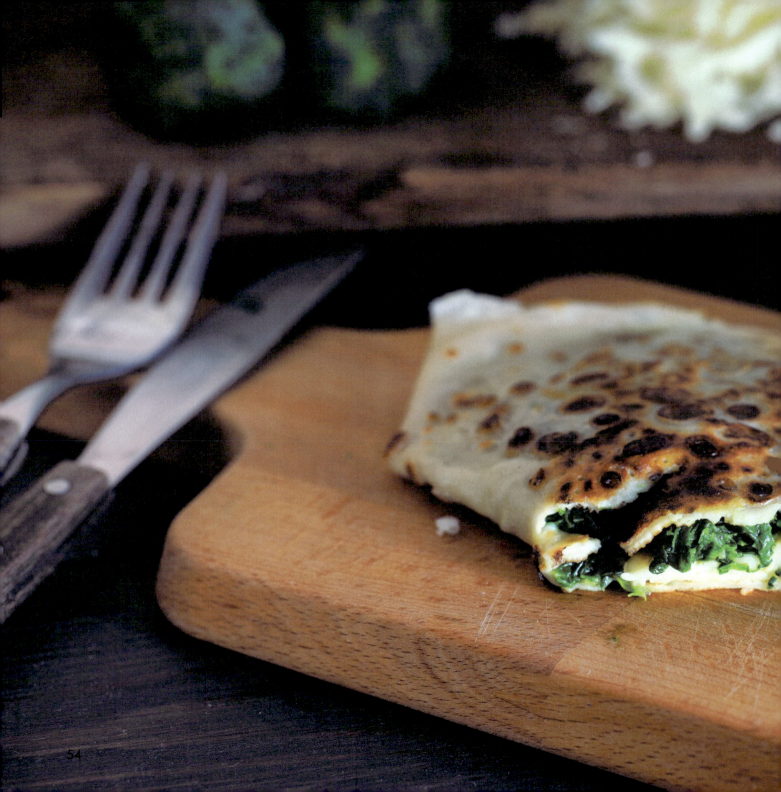

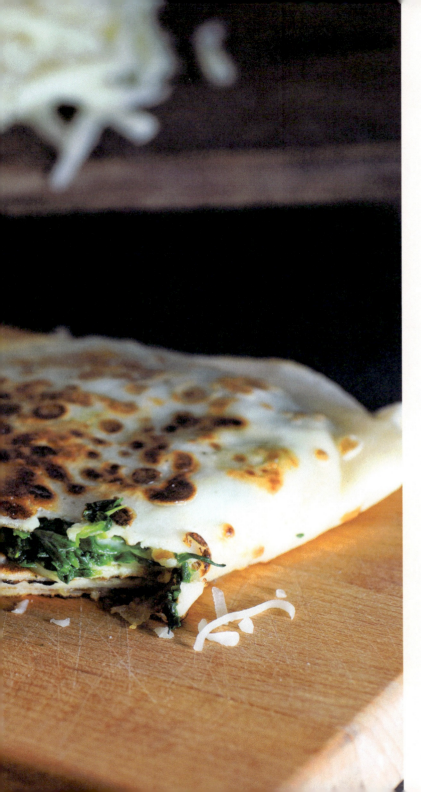

Savory Spinach Pancake

Ingredients

2 large eggs
1/8 teaspoon salt
½ teaspoon baking powder
½ teaspoon ground thyme
1 teaspoon ground cinnamon
1 teaspoon garlic/onion powder
1 teaspoon turmeric
¼ cup olive oil
1/3 cup all-purpose flour
½ cup frozen, chopped spinach
thawed and drained
Or ¾ cup chopped fresh spinach

Method

Beat eggs well.
Add salt and seasonings. Beat.
Add olive oil. Beat.
Mix in spinach.
Fold in flour and baking powder.
Thawed and drained spinach may
need an extra tablespoon of flour.
Cook pancakes in the usual way.

Makes 3 medium size pancakes.

Savory White Potato Pancake

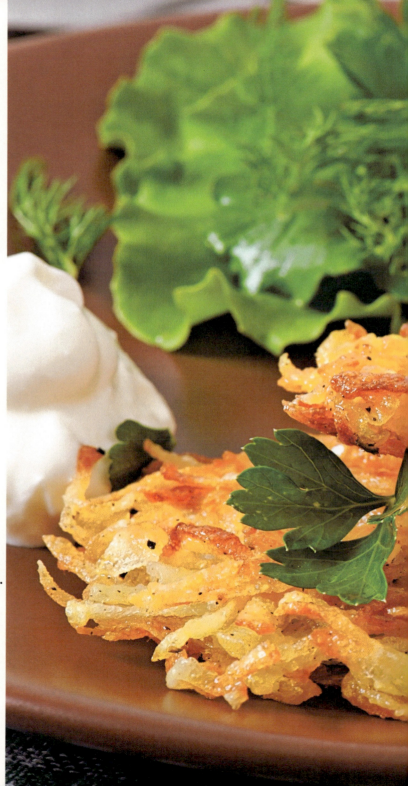

Ingredients

2 large eggs
1/8 teaspoon salt
½ teaspoon baking powder
½ teaspoon ground thyme
1 teaspoon ground cinnamon
1 teaspoon garlic/onion powder
1 teaspoon turmeric
¼ cup olive oil
¼ cup all-purpose flour
1 small white potato grated
or cooked and mashed

Method

Beat eggs well.
Add salt and seasonings. Beat.
Add olive oil. Beat.
Add cooked and mashed potato. Beat.
Or mix in grated potato.
Fold in flour and baking powder.
Cook pancakes in the usual way.

Makes 3 to 4 medium size pancakes.

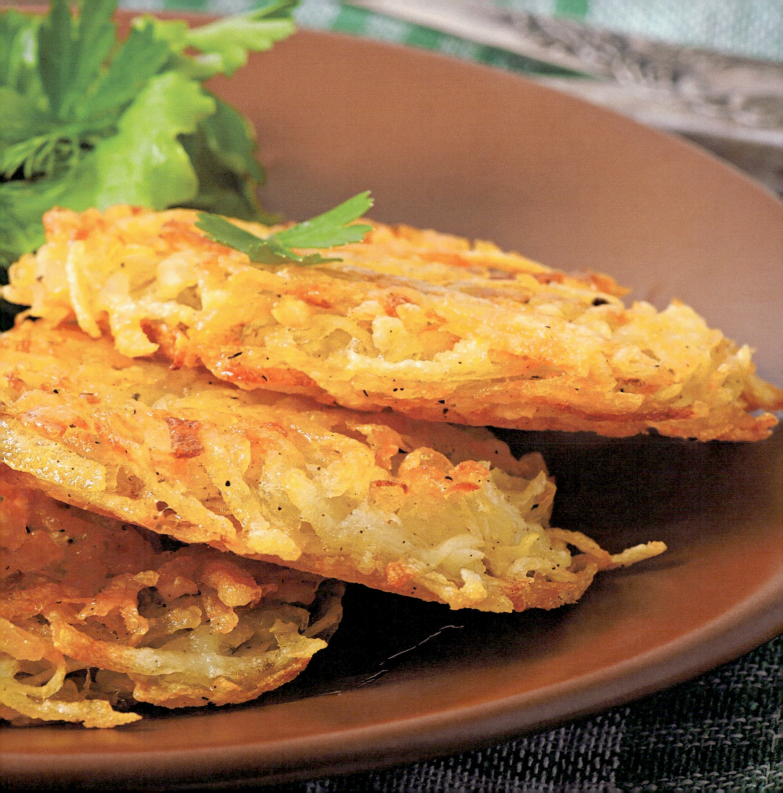

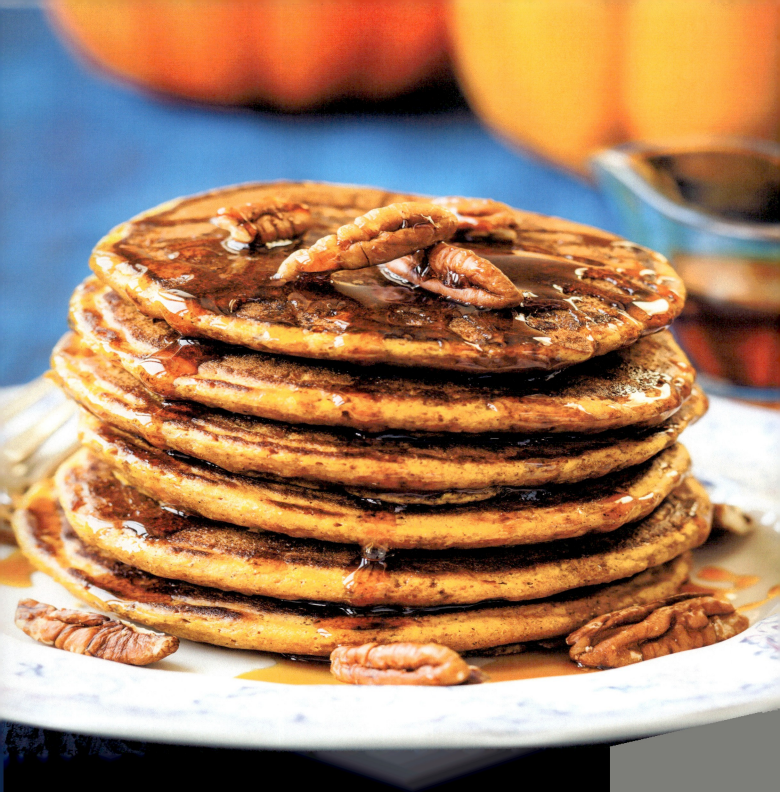

Savory Butternut Pancake

Ingredients

2 large eggs
1/8 teaspoon salt
½ teaspoon baking powder
½ teaspoon ground thyme
1 teaspoon ground cinnamon
1 teaspoon garlic/onion powder
1 teaspoon turmeric
¼ cup olive oil
1/3 cup all-purpose flour
½ cup cooked and mashed or ¾ cup grated butternut squash

Method

Beat eggs well.
Add salt and seasonings. Beat.
Add olive oil. Beat.
Add cooked and mashed butternut squash. Beat.
Or mix in grated butternut squash.
Fold in flour and baking powder.
Cook pancakes in the usual way.

Makes 3 to 4 medium size pancakes.

Savory Cheese Pancake

Ingredients

2 large eggs
A pinch of salt
½ teaspoon baking powder
½ teaspoon ground cinnamon
½ teaspoon garlic powder/
onion powder
½ teaspoon turmeric
¼ cup olive oil
1/3 cup cottage cheese or your
favorite shredded cheese
1/3 cup all-purpose flour

Method

Beat eggs well.
Add salt and seasonings. Beat.
Add olive oil. Beat.
Mix in cheese.
Fold in flour and baking powder.
Cook pancakes in the usual way.

Makes 3 medium size pancakes.

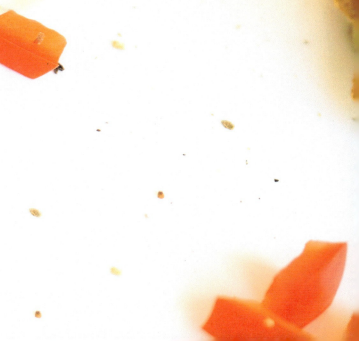

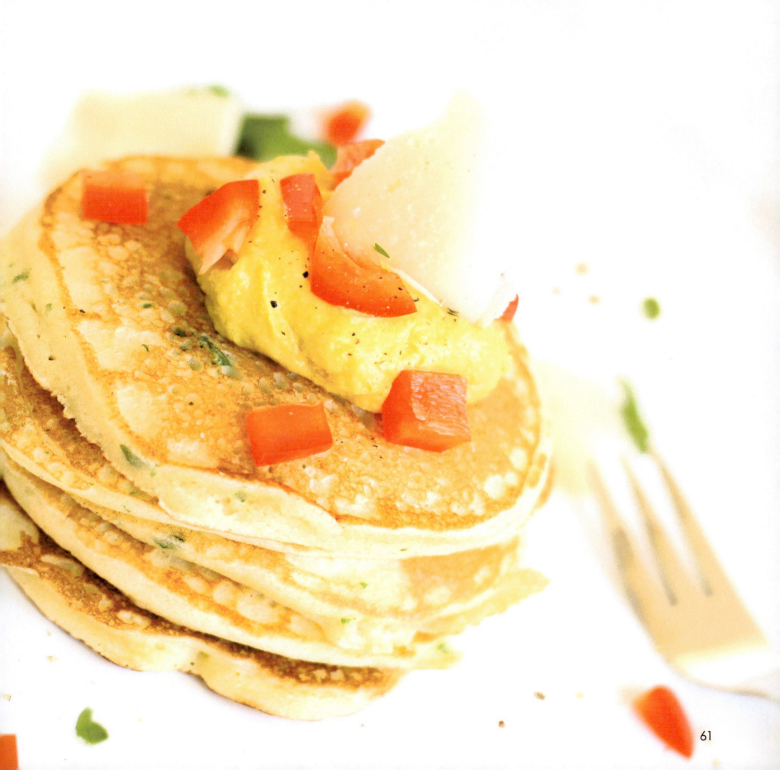